Preventing Dementia

Preventing Dementia

Karen L. Aken

ISBN-13: 978-1540747358
ISBN-10: 1540747352

Introduction

Loss of brain function is a scary thing. I remember after my Father watched my Grandfather slowly lose his mind and then his life to Alzheimer's he tried every way he could to not meet the same fate. He played a lot of Sudoku, tried to eat a healthier diet, and exercised daily. Sudoku seems to be the main exercise people go to when they fear dementia. Sudoku is great at exercising your brain, but it only exercises the brain's mathematical functions. If you are planning on doing lots of Math during your golden years, then doing Sudoku every day is perfect for you. If you would like to ensure that all of your brain's functions will continue to work properly, then you might want to add a wide variety of activities to improve all brain functions. The goal of this book is to change up your routine, help you start living a healthier lifestyle (if you aren't already), and to challenge your brain with new and sometimes random activities you may not have not done since you were a kid.

The information in this book is not intended or implied to be a substitute for professional medical advice, diagnosis or treatment. All content contained in this book is for general information purposes only. Any reliance you place on such information is therefore strictly at your own risk.

Day One

- Walk for at least 10 minutes this morning. Regular exercise can reduce your risk of Alzheimer's by 50% according to the Alzheimer's Research and Prevention Foundation.
- Drink seven glasses of water and two cups of green tea. Staying well hydrated ensures every organ in your body will function properly. Drinking Green Tea has been found to enhance memory and mental alertness and slow brain aging.
- Go to a quiet space, sit comfortably, close your eyes, take deep breaths and focus only on the air flowing into your nose, down into your lungs, and back out for 2 minutes. Meditation reduces stress which can have an adverse affect on the mind and body.
- Avoid slips, trips, and falls by improving your balance. Stand on one leg for 10 seconds, and then the other for 10 seconds.

Brain activities:

- While marching in place, think of the first house you lived in. How many bedrooms were there? How many bathrooms? What color was the kitchen? How many chairs were at your kitchen table? Can you remember the address? Can you remember the zip code? What was your favorite memory while there? This is your first Neuroplasticity exercise. Neuroplasticity is the brain's ability to change and adapt to new situations. Your brain would prefer to only perform one task at a time, this is why people turn down the radio to find an address or say they need to "stop and think for a minute". Answering simple questions while the body is in motion stresses the brain and forces it to improve much like traditional exercise forces your body to improve.
- Solve these problems in your head.

$11 \times 8 =$ ___ $6 + 32 =$ ___ $39 - 17 =$ ___ $12/3 =$ ___

Day Two

- Drink seven glasses of water and two cups of green tea.
- Walk for at least 10 minutes this morning.
- Go to a quiet space, sit comfortably, close your eyes, take deep breaths and focus only on the air flowing into your nose, down into your lungs, and back out for 2 minutes.
- Stand on one leg for 10 seconds, and then the other for 10 seconds.
- A Mediterranean diet has been found to reduce the risk of cognitive impairment and Alzheimer's. Research this diet. Say out loud the significant food sources involved with this diet. Vegetables, beans, whole grains, fish, and olive oil. Spell them (out loud) forwards and backwards. How often are these foods included in your diet?

Brain activities:

- Eat with your non-dominant hand today.
- Solve these problems in your head.

$6 \times 7 =$ ___ $43 + 18 =$ ___ $74 - 6 =$ ___ $32/8 =$ ___

- Name 3 States that begin with the letter I.
- What movie makes you laugh the most? Why?

Day Three

- ☐ Drink seven glasses of water and two cups of green tea.
- ☐ Walk for at least 10 minutes this morning.
- ☐ Go to a quiet space, sit comfortably, close your eyes, take deep breaths and focus only on the air flowing into your nose, down into your lungs, and back out for 2 minutes.
- ☐ Stand on one leg for 10 seconds, and then the other for 10 seconds.

Brain activities:

- ☐ Learn to juggle with juggling scarves or handkerchiefs (instructions on next page). German researchers have found that learning to juggle increases grey matter in the brain in as little as 7 days. Once you know how, turn this into an advanced Neuroplasticity exercise by singing the alphabet or your favorite song while juggling or walking forwards or backwards while juggling.
- ☐ Solve these problems in your head.

13 x 2 = ____   57 + 8 = ____   64 - 6 = ____   64/8 = ____

- ☐ Name 3 of the Seven Dwarfs.
- ☐ What was your favorite book to read as a child? What was it about?

Juggling with scarves or handkerchiefs (actual juggling scarves work better).

1 scarf - Hold the scarf at one corner. Lift your arm as high as you can across your body, and toss the scarf with the palm of your hand facing outwards (like you are waving goodbye to someone). Reach high up with your other hand and catch the scarf as you bring your hand down. Repeat this move and throw back to the first hand. Try to make each throw to the same height (peak).

2 scarves - Hold a scarf in each hand. Throw a scarf from one hand. When it reaches its peak, throw the second scarf. Then catch the first scarf, then the second. The throws and catches should be in rhythm (throw, throw, catch, catch). Don't throw or catch both scarves at the same time.

3 scarves - Two scarves in your dominant hand (holding one with your pinky and ring finger, and one with your middle and forefinger) and one scarf in your non-dominant hand. Throw one scarf from your dominant hand, when it reaches its peak, throw the scarf from your non-dominant hand. When that scarf reaches its peak, you can throw the third scarf, and then just keep alternating throws between hands.

Day Four

- Drink seven glasses of water and two cups of green tea.
- Walk for at least 10 minutes this morning.
- Go to a quiet space, sit comfortably, close your eyes, take deep breaths and focus only on the air flowing into your nose, down into your lungs, and back out for 2 minutes.
- Stand on one leg for 10 seconds, and then the other for 10 seconds.

Brain activities:

- Alternate moving one side of your body with the other (ex. lunges, leg kicks or tap your toes) while clapping your hands. Say a different animal every time you move the right side of your body. Say a place you have been or would like to travel every time you move the left side. Perform this Neuroplasticity exercise for at least one minute.
- Solve these problems in your head.

  44 x 3 = ____   19 + 83 = ____   25 - 13 = ____   45/9 = ____
- Name 3 animals that begin with the letter D.
- Who was your first boss? Describe what he or she looked like out loud.
- Open cupboards and drawers without using your fingers today.

Day Five

- Drink seven glasses of water and two cups of green tea.
- Walk for at least 10 minutes this morning.
- Go to a quiet space, sit comfortably, close your eyes, take deep breaths and focus only on the air flowing into your nose, down into your lungs, and back out for 2 minutes.
- Stand on one leg for 10 seconds, and then the other for 10 seconds.

Brain activities:

- While marching in place and clapping your hands, say out loud the 12 months of the year. Spell them forward. Spell them backward. How many months are typically hot? How many months are typically cold? Which month gets the most rain? Which month gets the least?
- Brush your teeth with your non-dominant hand today.
- Solve these problems in your head.

$15 \times 2 =$ ___ $28 + 42 =$ ___ $99 - 23 =$ ___ $72/12 =$ ___

- Name 3 foods that begin with the letter L.
- What was the name of the street you lived on when you were in high school? Picture your route to school. How long did it take you to get there from home?

Day Six

- Drink seven glasses of water and two cups of green tea.
- Walk for at least 10 minutes this morning.
- Go to a quiet space, sit comfortably, close your eyes, take deep breaths and focus only on the air flowing into your nose, down into your lungs, and back out for 2 minutes.
- To improve balance, stand on one leg for 10 seconds, and then the other for 10 seconds.

Brain activities:

- Put your hands together. Move your hands in a figure 8 motion in front of your body while marching in place. While your body is in motion, say your favorite fruit out loud. Spell it forward. Spell it backward. How many letters does the word have? Does your telephone number contain that number? If yes, say the section of your phone number that contains that number. Repeat the answer backwards. If no, repeat any section of your phone number backwards. This Neuroplasticity exercise should be done with a partner who can ask you the questions.
- Solve these problems in your head.

$51 \times 2 =$ ___ $55 + 31 =$ ___ $49 - 33 =$ ___ $22/2 =$ ___

- Name 3 plants that begin with the letter R.
- What did you eat for dinner last night? What did you eat for lunch 2 days ago?

Day Seven

- Drink seven glasses of water and two cups of green tea.
- Walk for at least 10 minutes this morning.
- Go to a quiet space, sit comfortably, close your eyes, take deep breaths and focus only on the air flowing into your nose, down into your lungs, and back out for 2 minutes.
- To improve balance, stand on one leg for 10 seconds, and then the other for 10 seconds.

Brain activities:

- March in place while rubbing your belly in a circular motion with your dominant hand, alternate touching your left and right ears with your non-dominate hand while singing the alphabet.
- Solve these problems in your head.

$84 \times 4 =$ ___ $39 + 14 =$ ___ $104 - 26 =$ ___ $120/10 =$ ___

- Name 3 actors/actresses whose names that begin with the letter T.
- Without looking at the calendar, what were the last 2 holidays and what are the next 2? What did you do for the last 2 holidays? What will you do for the next?

Day Eight

- Drink seven glasses of water and three cups of green tea. Just a reminder, staying well hydrated ensures every organ in your body will function properly. Drinking Green Tea has been found to enhance memory and mental alertness and slow brain aging.
- Walk for at least 10 minutes this morning and 10 minutes this afternoon. Just a reminder, regular exercise can reduce your risk of Alzheimer's by 50% according to the Alzheimer's Research and Prevention Foundation.
- Go to a quiet space, sit comfortably, close your eyes, take deep breaths and focus only on the air flowing into your nose, down into your lungs, and back out for 3 minutes. Just a reminder, meditation reduces stress which can have an adverse affect on the mind and body.
- To improve balance, stand on one leg for 10 seconds, and then the other for 10 seconds.

Brain activities:

- While marching in place and doing arm circles, think of your high school. Around how many people were in your graduation class? How many floors did the school have? Can you remember who your favorite teacher was? Where was the lunch room? Where was the gym? Can you remember your favorite class? What was your favorite memory while there?
- Solve these problems in your head.

$12 \times 9 = \underline{\quad}$ $7 + 43 = \underline{\quad}$ $40 - 18 = \underline{\quad}$ $13/1 = \underline{\quad}$

- Name 3 cities that begin with the letter A.

Day Nine

- Drink seven glasses of water and three cups of green tea.
- Walk for at least 10 minutes this morning and 10 minutes this afternoon.
- Go to a quiet space, sit comfortably, close your eyes, take deep breaths and focus only on the air flowing into your nose, down into your lungs, and back out for 3 minutes.
- Stand on one leg for 10 seconds, and then the other for 10 seconds.

Brain activities:

- Eat with your non-dominant hand today.
- Solve these problems in your head.

$7 \times 8 =$ ___ $54 + 29 =$ ___ $85 - 7 =$ ___ $44/2 =$ ___

- Spell out loud 3 girls names that begin with the letter C.
- What comedian makes you laugh the most? Describe the way they look out loud.

Day Ten

- Drink seven glasses of water and three cups of green tea.
- Walk for at least 10 minutes this morning and 10 minutes this afternoon.
- Go to a quiet space, sit comfortably, close your eyes, take deep breaths and focus only on the air flowing into your nose, down into your lungs, and back out for 3 minutes.
- Stand on one leg for 10 seconds, and then the other for 10 seconds.

Brain activities:

- Juggle with scarves. Just a reminder, German researchers have found that learning to juggle increases grey matter in the brain in as little as 7 days. Once you know how, sing the alphabet or your favorite song while juggling or walk forwards or backwards while juggling to turn this into an advanced Neuroplasticity exercise.
- Solve these problems in your head.

24 x 3 = ___   68 + 9 = ___   76 - 7 = ___   75/5 = ___

- Name the 3 states that start with the letter C.
- What was your favorite food to eat as a child? How often did you eat it?
- Brush your teeth with your non-dominant hand today.

Day Eleven

- Drink seven glasses of water and three cups of green tea.
- Walk for at least 10 minutes this morning and 10 minutes this afternoon.
- Go to a quiet space, sit comfortably, close your eyes, take deep breaths and focus only on the air flowing into your nose, down into your lungs, and back out for 3 minutes.
- Stand on one leg for 10 seconds, and then the other for 10 seconds.

Brain activities:

- Alternate moving one side of your body with the other (ex. lunges, leg kicks or tap your toes) while clapping your hands. Say a different fruit every time you move the right side of your body. Say a different vegetable every time you move the left side. Perform this exercise for at least one minute.
- Solve these problems in your head.

$55 \times 3 =$ ___ $20 + 94 =$ ___ $66 - 14 =$ ___ $54/9 =$ ___

- Name 3 animals that begin with the letter S.
- Who was your first crush? What did they look like?

Day Twelve

- Drink seven glasses of water and three cups of green tea.
- Walk for at least 10 minutes this morning and 10 minutes this afternoon.
- Go to a quiet space, sit comfortably, close your eyes, take deep breaths and focus only on the air flowing into your nose, down into your lungs, and back out for 3 minutes.
- Stand on one leg for 10 seconds, and then the other for 10 seconds.

Brain activities:

- Brush your teeth with your non-dominant hand.
- Solve these problems in your head.

61 x 2 = ___   93 + 25 = ___   90 - 33 = ___   48/4= ___

- Name 5 condiments.
- What was the name of your best friend when you were in elementary school? What did they look like? What was your favorite thing to do with them?

Day Thirteen

- Drink seven glasses of water and three cups of green tea.
- Walk for at least 10 minutes this morning and 10 minutes this afternoon.
- Go to a quiet space, sit comfortably, close your eyes, take deep breaths and focus only on the air flowing into your nose, down into your lungs, and back out for 3 minutes.
- Stand on one leg for 10 seconds, and then the other for 10 seconds.

Brain activities:

- Put your hands together. Move your hands in a figure 8 motion in front of your body while marching in place. While your body is in motion, say your favorite animal out loud. Spell it forward. Spell it backward. How many letters does the word have? Does your telephone number contain that number? If yes, say the section of your phone number that contains that number. Repeat the answer backwards. If no, repeat any section of your phone number backwards. This exercise should be done with a partner who can ask you the questions.
- Solve these problems in your head.

$15 \times 2 =$ ___ $55 + 13 =$ ___ $94 - 36 =$ ___ $57/3 =$ ___

- Name 3 plants that begin with the letter P.
- What did you eat for dinner two days ago? What did you eat for breakfast 3 days ago?

Day Fourteen

- Drink seven glasses of water and three cups of green tea.
- Walk for at least 10 minutes this morning and 10 minutes this afternoon.
- Go to a quiet space, sit comfortably, close your eyes, take deep breaths and focus only on the air flowing into your nose, down into your lungs, and back out for 3 minutes.
- Stand on one leg for 10 seconds, and then the other for 10 seconds.

Brain activities:

- March in place while rubbing your belly in a circular motion with your dominant hand, alternate touching your left and right ears with your non-dominant hand while singing the alphabet.
- Solve these problems in your head.

85 x 2 = ___   94 + 15 = ___   62 - 40 = ___   86/2 = ___

- Name 3 politicians past or present with first or last names that begin with the letter T.
- How many people do you know were born in November? Say and spell their names out loud.

Day Fifteen

- Drink seven glasses of water and three cups of green tea.
- Walk for at least 10 minutes this morning and 10 minutes this afternoon.
- Go to a quiet space, sit comfortably, close your eyes, take deep breaths and focus only on the air flowing into your nose, down into your lungs, and back out for 3 minutes.
- Stand on one leg for 10 seconds, and then the other for 10 seconds.

Brain activities:

- While marching in place and doing arm circles at the same time, think of a day you spent at an amusement park or zoo. How many people went with you? How long ago did you go? What was the weather like the day you went? Was it a long line to get in? What was your favorite moment while there?
- Joe has a $500 deductible. If he has already paid $305 in October and $90 in November, how much more does he need to pay to meet the deductible?
- Brush your teeth with your non-dominant hand today.
- Name 3 cities that begin with the letter H.

Day Sixteen

- Drink seven glasses of water and three cups of green tea.
- Walk for at least 10 minutes this morning and 10 minutes this afternoon.
- Go to a quiet space, sit comfortably, close your eyes, take deep breaths and focus only on the air flowing into your nose, down into your lungs, and back out for 3 minutes.
- Stand on one leg for 10 seconds, and then the other for 10 seconds.

Brain activities:

- Eat with your non-dominant hand today.
- There are 60 flowers in the garden. They are arranged in rows that have 5 daisies and 5 tulips each. How many rows of flowers are in the garden?
- Spell 3 holidays out loud forwards and backwards.
- Name at least 3 snacks available at movie theaters besides popcorn.
- Open cupboards and drawers without using your fingers today.

Day Seventeen

- Drink seven glasses of water and three cups of green tea.
- Walk for at least 10 minutes this morning and 10 minutes this afternoon.
- Go to a quiet space, sit comfortably, close your eyes, take deep breaths and focus only on the air flowing into your nose, down into your lungs, and back out for 3 minutes.
- Stand on one leg for 10 seconds, and then the other for 10 seconds.

Brain activities:

- Juggle with scarves today while singing Happy Birthday, the alphabet, or your national anthem.
- Lucy has 52 gnomes in her front yard. Her neighbor Bob hates gnomes. Bob shoots 18 of them with his rifle while Lucy is out of town. How many gnomes does Lucy have left? The gnomes cost $15 each. How much will Lucy need to charge Bob to replace the gnomes?
- Name 3 states that begin with the letter A.
- What was your favorite game to play as a child? Who would play with you?

Day Eighteen

- Drink seven glasses of water and three cups of green tea.
- Walk for at least 10 minutes this morning and 10 minutes this afternoon.
- Go to a quiet space, sit comfortably, close your eyes, take deep breaths and focus only on the air flowing into your nose, down into your lungs, and back out for 3 minutes.
- Stand on one leg for 10 seconds, and then the other for 10 seconds.

Brain activities:

- Alternate moving one side of your body with the other (ex. lunges, leg kicks or tap your toes) while clapping your hands. Say a different city every time you move the right side of your body. Say a different state every time you move the left side. Perform this exercise for at least one minute.
- Judy likes to get her hair done at least once a month. Her hair stylist usually charges Judy $24 per style. When her stylist does well, Judy tips her 20%. When her stylist does bad, Judy tips her 15%. Her stylist was having a really bad day. Judy now looks just like her toy poodle. An 8% tip will be how much?
- Name 3 animals that begin with the letter M.
- Who were your first neighbors? Was it a family? If so, how many people were there and what were there names?

Day Nineteen

- Drink seven glasses of water and three cups of green tea.
- Walk for at least 10 minutes this morning and 10 minutes this afternoon.
- Go to a quiet space, sit comfortably, close your eyes, take deep breaths and focus only on the air flowing into your nose, down into your lungs, and back out for 3 minutes.
- Stand on one leg for 10 seconds, and then the other for 10 seconds.

Brain activities:

- Brush your teeth with your non-dominant hand.
- Ruth tried to teach her granddaughter Hailey how to bake cookies. Together they made 24 snickerdoodles, 26 sugar cookies, and 27 pumpkin cookies. 1/3 of them were burnt to a crisp. How many edible cookies were there?
- Name 3 foods that begin with the letter W.
- What is your favorite song? Write down your favorite verse and count how many letters are in the sentence. How many T's are there? How many E's? How many A's? How many S's?

Day Twenty

- Drink seven glasses of water and three cups of green tea.
- Walk for at least 10 minutes this morning and 10 minutes this afternoon.
- Go to a quiet space, sit comfortably, close your eyes, take deep breaths and focus only on the air flowing into your nose, down into your lungs, and back out for 3 minutes.
- Stand on one leg for 10 seconds, and then the other for 10 seconds.

Brain activities:

- Put your hands together. Move your hands in a figure 8 motion in front of your body while marching in place. While your body is in motion, say your favorite city out loud. Spell it forward. Spell it backward. How many letters does the word have? Does your telephone number contain that number? If yes, say the section of your phone number that contains that number. Repeat the answer backwards. If no, repeat any section of your phone number backwards. This exercise should be done with a partner who can ask you the questions.
- Karen tries to teach her daughter Mercedes how to drive. If they drive 112 miles at a 35 mph pace, how long will Karen be pulling her hair out and biting her nails for?
- Spell out loud 3 boys names that begin with the letter C.
- What did you eat for lunch two days ago? What did you eat for dinner four days ago?

Day Twenty-One

- Drink seven glasses of water and three cups of green tea.
- Walk for at least 10 minutes this morning and 10 minutes this afternoon.
- Go to a quiet space, sit comfortably, close your eyes, take deep breaths and focus only on the air flowing into your nose, down into your lungs, and back out for 3 minutes.
- Stand on one leg for 10 seconds, and then the other for 10 seconds.

Brain activities:

- March in place while rubbing your belly in a circular motion with your dominant hand, alternate touching your left and right ears with your non-dominant hand while singing the alphabet backwards.
- Gary likes to check out garage sales in the neighborhood. If he spent $2.50 on a tool he doesn't need, $3.35 on an old record he forgot he already had, and $0.75 on a flashlight that won't work for very long, how much of his $20 did he waste?
- Name 3 magazines that people used to read in print.
- How many months until the end of the year? How many weeks? How many days?

Day Twenty-two

- ☐ Drink seven glasses of water and three cups of green tea.
- ☐ Walk for at least 15 minutes this morning and 15 minutes this afternoon.
- ☐ Go to a quiet space, sit comfortably, close your eyes, take deep breaths and focus only on the air flowing into your nose, down into your lungs, and back out for 4 minutes.
- ☐ Stand on one leg for 15 seconds, and then the other for 15 seconds.

Brain activities:

- ☐ While marching in place and doing arm circles, think of your first job. How many people worked there? What hours did you work? Did you wear a uniform? If so, what did it look like? Which co-worker did you like the most? Which co-worker did you like the least?
- ☐ Solve these problems in your head.

23 x 6 = ____   11 + 79 = ____   78 - 24 = ____   45/9 = ____

- ☐ How many words can you make with the following letters:

                    A D N L O
- ☐ Name 3 cities that begin with the letter O.
- ☐ Work on memorizing the fifty United States this week.

Alabama	Colorado
Alaska	Connecticut
Arizona	Delaware
Arkansas	Florida
California	Georgia

Day Twenty-three

- Drink seven glasses of water and three cups of green tea.
- Walk for at least 15 minutes this morning and 15 minutes this afternoon.
- Go to a quiet space, sit comfortably, close your eyes, take deep breaths and focus only on the air flowing into your nose, down into your lungs, and back out for 4 minutes.
- Stand on one leg for 15 seconds, and then the other for 15 seconds.

Brain activities:

- Eat with your non-dominant hand today.
- Solve these problems in your head.

$77 \times 8 =$ ___ $154 + 92 =$ ___ $185 - 72 =$ ___ $144/2 =$ ___

- How many words can you make with the following letters:

R P S A E

- Say and spell all of the days of the week out loud.
- Read everything out loud today.
- Work on memorizing the fifty United States this week.

Hawaii	Kansas
Idaho	Kentucky
Illinois	Louisiana
Indiana	Maine
Iowa	Maryland

Day Twenty-four

- Drink seven glasses of water and three cups of green tea.
- Walk for at least 15 minutes this morning and 15 minutes this afternoon.
- Go to a quiet space, sit comfortably, close your eyes, take deep breaths and focus only on the air flowing into your nose, down into your lungs, and back out for 4 minutes.
- Stand on one leg for 15 seconds, and then the other for 15 seconds.

Brain activities:

- Time to juggle with scarves. Count each time you throw a scarf. How high can you get?
- Solve these problems in your head.

$35 \times 4 =$ ___ $168 + 19 =$ ___ $761 - 171 =$ ___ $95/5 =$ ___

- How many words can you make with the following letters:

CTINH

- Name the 3 states that begin with the letter W.
- When you were a kid what did you want to be when you grew up?
- Work on memorizing the fifty United States this week.

Massachusetts	Montana
Michigan	Nebraska
Minnesota	Nevada
Mississippi	New Hampshire
Missouri	New Jersey

Day Twenty-five

- Drink seven glasses of water and three cups of green tea.
- Walk for at least 15 minutes this morning and 15 minutes this afternoon.
- Go to a quiet space, sit comfortably, close your eyes, take deep breaths and focus only on the air flowing into your nose, down into your lungs, and back out for 4 minutes.
- Stand on one leg for 15 seconds, and then the other for 15 seconds.

Brain activities:

- Alternate moving one side of your body with the other (ex. lunges, leg kicks or tap your toes) while clapping your hands. Say a different letter every time you move the right side of your body. Say a different number every time you move the left side. Perform this exercise for at least one minute.
- Solve these problems in your head.

$50 \times 13 = $ ___ $120 + 941 = $ ___ $166 - 148 = $ ___ $52/4 = $ ___

- How many words can you make with the following letters:

W L A H E

- Work on memorizing the fifty United States this week.

New Mexico	Oklahoma
New York	Oregon
North Carolina	Pennsylvania
North Dakota	Rhode Island
Ohio	South Carolina

Day Twenty-six

- Drink seven glasses of water and three cups of green tea.
- Walk for at least 15 minutes this morning and 15 minutes this afternoon.
- Go to a quiet space, sit comfortably, close your eyes, take deep breaths and focus only on the air flowing into your nose, down into your lungs, and back out for 4 minutes.
- Stand on one leg for 15 seconds, and then the other for 15 seconds.

Brain activities:

- Brush your teeth with your non-dominant hand.
- Solve these problems in your head.

$16 \times 6 =$ ___ $183 + 52 =$ ___ $901 - 33 =$ ___ $138/6 =$ ___

- How many words can you make with the following letters:

U B L R E

- Name 3 trees. Do any of them change color in the fall? If so, what colors?
- When did you stop believing in Santa? The tooth fairy? How did you feel when you found out the truth?
- Work on memorizing the fifty United States this week.

South Dakota	Virginia
Tennessee	Washington
Texas	West Virginia
Utah	Wisconsin
Vermont	Wyoming

Day Twenty-seven

- Drink seven glasses of water and three cups of green tea.
- Walk for at least 15 minutes this morning and 15 minutes this afternoon.
- Go to a quiet space, sit comfortably, close your eyes, take deep breaths and focus only on the air flowing into your nose, down into your lungs, and back out for 4 minutes.
- Stand on one leg for 15 seconds, and then the other for 15 seconds.

Brain activities:

- Put your hands together. Move your hands in a figure 8 motion in front of your body while marching in place. While your body is in motion, say your favorite holiday out loud. Spell it forward. Spell it backward. How many letters does the word have? Does your telephone number contain that number? If yes, say the section of your phone number that contains that number. Repeat the answer backwards. If no, repeat any section of your phone number backwards. This exercise should be done with a partner who can ask you the questions.
- Solve these problems in your head.

$151 \times 2 = $ ___ $551 + 131 = $ ___ $63 - 49 = $ ___ $288 / 12 = $ ___

- How many words can you make with the following letters:

A D O R I

- Name 3 oceans and 3 lakes. Where are they located?
- What did you eat for dinner three days ago? What did you eat for lunch two days ago?
- Continue to work on memorizing the fifty United States.

Day Twenty-eight

- Drink seven glasses of water and three cups of green tea.
- Walk for at least 15 minutes this morning and 15 minutes this afternoon.
- Go to a quiet space, sit comfortably, close your eyes, take deep breaths and focus only on the air flowing into your nose, down into your lungs, and back out for 4 minutes.
- Stand on one leg for 15 seconds, and then the other for 15 seconds.

Brain activities:

- March in place while rubbing your belly in a circular motion with your dominant hand, alternate touching your left and right ears with your non-dominant hand while singing your national anthem.
- Solve these problems in your head.

  $58 \times 3 =$ ___ $641 + 263 =$ ___ $621 - 408 =$ ___ $96/3 =$ ___
- How many words can you make with the following letters:

  B I M C E
- Name 3 politicians past or present with first or last names that start with the letter G.
- How many people do you know were born in August?
- Continue to work on memorizing the fifty United States.

Day Twenty-nine

- Drink seven glasses of water and three cups of green tea.
- Walk for at least 15 minutes this morning and 15 minutes this afternoon.
- Go to a quiet space, sit comfortably, close your eyes, take deep breaths and focus only on the air flowing into your nose, down into your lungs, and back out for 4 minutes.
- Stand on one leg for 15 seconds, and then the other for 15 seconds.

Brain activities:

- While marching in place and doing arm circles, think of the first home you lived in. How many bedrooms were there? How many bathrooms? What color was the kitchen? How many chairs were at your kitchen table? Can you remember the address? Can you remember the zip code? What was your favorite memory while there?
- Rearrange items in your kitchen to alter your routine. This will help your brain create new neural pathways.
- Name 3 cities that begin with the letter N.

Day Thirty

- Drink seven glasses of water and three cups of green tea.
- Walk for at least 15 minutes this morning and 15 minutes this afternoon.
- Go to a quiet space, sit comfortably, close your eyes, take deep breaths and focus only on the air flowing into your nose, down into your lungs, and back out for 4 minutes.
- Stand on one leg for 15 seconds, and then the other for 15 seconds.

Brain activities:

- Eat with your non-dominant hand today.
- Using a pencil and paper, draw a dog, a house, and a car with your dominant hand. Then draw the same pictures with your non-dominant hand.
- Name 3 States that begin with the letter W.
- What was your favorite movie when you were a child? Can you remember any of the actors/actresses that were in it?

Day Thirty-one

- Drink seven glasses of water and three cups of green tea.
- Walk for at least 15 minutes this morning and 15 minutes this afternoon.
- Go to a quiet space, sit comfortably, close your eyes, take deep breaths and focus only on the air flowing into your nose, down into your lungs, and back out for 4 minutes.
- Stand on one leg for 15 seconds, and then the other for 15 seconds.

Brain activities:

- Sing the alphabet or your favorite song while juggling or walk forwards or backwards while juggling.
- Rearrange items in your bathroom to alter your routine. This will help your brain create new neural pathways.
- Name 3 types of seasoning that you never use.
- If there is a chair that you always sit in, choose another seat for the next three days and avoid your normal one.

Day Thirty-two

- Drink seven glasses of water and three cups of green tea.
- Walk for at least 15 minutes this morning and 15 minutes this afternoon.
- Go to a quiet space, sit comfortably, close your eyes, take deep breaths and focus only on the air flowing into your nose, down into your lungs, and back out for 4 minutes.
- Stand on one leg for 15 seconds, and then the other for 15 seconds.

Brain activities:

- Alternate moving one side of your body with the other (ex. lunges, leg kicks or tap your toes) while clapping your hands. Say a different animal every time you move the right side of your body. Say a place you have been or would like to travel every time you move the left side. Perform this exercise for at least one minute.
- Just a reminder, a Mediterranean diet has been found to reduce the risk of cognitive impairment and Alzheimer's. Say out loud the significant food sources involved with this diet. Vegetables, beans, whole grains, fish, and olive oil. Spell them (out loud) forwards and backwards. How often are these foods included in your diet?
- Name 3 animals that begin with the letter B.

Day Thirty-three

- Drink seven glasses of water and three cups of green tea.
- Walk for at least 15 minutes this morning and 15 minutes this afternoon.
- Go to a quiet space, sit comfortably, close your eyes, take deep breaths and focus only on the air flowing into your nose, down into your lungs, and back out for 4 minutes.
- Stand on one leg for 15 seconds, and then the other for 15 seconds.

Brain activities:

- Brush your teeth with your non-dominant hand.
- Rearrange items in your closet to alter your routine. This will help your brain create new neural pathways.
- Name 6 foods that begin with the letter B.
- What was the name of the street you lived on when you were 20?

Day Thirty-four

- Drink seven glasses of water and three cups of green tea.
- Walk for at least 15 minutes this morning and 15 minutes this afternoon.
- Go to a quiet space, sit comfortably, close your eyes, take deep breaths and focus only on the air flowing into your nose, down into your lungs, and back out for 4 minutes.
- Stand on one leg for 15 seconds, and then the other for 15 seconds.

Brain activities:

- Put your hands together. Move your hands in a figure 8 motion in front of your body while marching in place. While your body is in motion, say your favorite fruit out loud. Spell it forward. Spell it backward. How many letters does the word have? Does your telephone number contain that number? If yes, say the section of your phone number that contains that number. Repeat the answer backwards. If no, repeat any section of your phone number backwards. This exercise should be done with a partner who can ask you the questions.
- Using a pencil and paper, draw a cat, a school, and a bicycle with your dominant hand. Then draw the same pictures with your non-dominant hand.

Day Thirty-five

- Drink seven glasses of water and three cups of green tea.
- Walk for at least 15 minutes this morning and 15 minutes this afternoon.
- Go to a quiet space, sit comfortably, close your eyes, take deep breaths and focus only on the air flowing into your nose, down into your lungs, and back out for 4 minutes.
- Stand on one leg for 15 seconds, and then the other for 15 seconds.

Brain activities:

- March in place while rubbing your belly in a circular motion with your dominant hand, alternate touching your left and right ears with your non-dominant hand while singing the alphabet.
- Make a paper airplane. Take a piece of paper. Fold it in half, lengthwise. Fold the top corners toward the center. Fold the angled edges toward the center. Fold along the center crease. Fold down the top two flaps to make the wings.
- Brush your teeth with your non-dominant hand today.

Day Thirty-six

- Drink seven glasses of water and three cups of green tea.
- Walk for at least 15 minutes this morning and 15 minutes this afternoon.
- Go to a quiet space, sit comfortably, close your eyes, take deep breaths and focus only on the air flowing into your nose, down into your lungs, and back out for 5 minutes.
- Stand on one leg for 15 seconds, and then the other for 15 seconds.

Brain activities:

- While marching in place and doing arm circles, think of your family. How many aunts and uncles do you have? Where do/did they live? Say their names out loud. How many cousins do you have? Where do/did they live? Say their names out loud. What memories do you have of time spent with them?
- Make a list of either grocery items, things to do, or anything else that comes to mind and memorize it. In an hour or so, see how many items you can recall. Make the items on your list as challenging as possible for the greatest mental stimulation.

Day Thirty-seven

- Drink seven glasses of water and three cups of green tea.
- Walk for at least 15 minutes this morning and 15 minutes this afternoon.
- Go to a quiet space, sit comfortably, close your eyes, take deep breaths and focus only on the air flowing into your nose, down into your lungs, and back out for 5 minutes.
- Stand on one leg for 15 seconds, and then the other for 15 seconds.

Brain activities:

- Eat with your non-dominant hand today.

Answer the following riddles:

- You can always find me in the past. I can be created in the present, but the future can never taint me. What am I?
- What belongs to you, but others use it more than you do?
- The more you take, the more you leave behind?

Answers at the bottom of day thirty-nine.

Day Thirty-eight

- Drink seven glasses of water and three cups of green tea.
- Walk for at least 15 minutes this morning and 15 minutes this afternoon.
- Go to a quiet space, sit comfortably, close your eyes, take deep breaths and focus only on the air flowing into your nose, down into your lungs, and back out for 5 minutes.
- Stand on one leg for 15 seconds, and then the other for 15 seconds.

Brain activities:

- Juggle with scarves. Sing Humpty Dumpty or your favorite song while juggling or walk forwards or backwards.
- Solve these problems in your head.

$2 + 3 + 4 + 5 + 5 =$ ___ $76 - 9 - 8 - 7 - 2 - 1 =$ ___

- Draw a bird, plate of food, and an angel with your dominant hand. Now draw the same pictures with your non-dominant hand.
- Open cupboards and drawers without using your fingers today.

Day Thirty-nine

- Drink seven glasses of water and three cups of green tea.
- Walk for at least 15 minutes this morning and 15 minutes this afternoon.
- Go to a quiet space, sit comfortably, close your eyes, take deep breaths and focus only on the air flowing into your nose, down into your lungs, and back out for 5 minutes.
- Stand on one leg for 15 seconds, and then the other for 15 seconds.

Brain activities:

- Alternate moving one side of your body with the other (ex. lunges, leg kicks or tap your toes) while clapping your hands. Say a different fruit every time you move the right side of your body. Say a different vegetable every time you move the left side. Perform this exercise for at least one minute.
- Solve these problems in your head.

$33 \times 6 =$ ___ $22 + 83 =$ ___ $176 - 41 =$ ___ $99/9 =$ ___

- Write a short story.

(A) History, Your Name, Footsteps

Day Forty

- Drink seven glasses of water and three cups of green tea.
- Walk for at least 15 minutes this morning and 15 minutes this afternoon.
- Go to a quiet space, sit comfortably, close your eyes, take deep breaths and focus only on the air flowing into your nose, down into your lungs, and back out for 5 minutes.
- Stand on one leg for 15 seconds, and then the other for 15 seconds.

Brain activities:

- Brush your teeth with your non-dominant hand.
- Solve these problems in your head.

$93 \times 2 =$ ___ $33 + 25 =$ ___ $48 - 33 =$ ___ $112/4 =$ ___

- Get a coloring book and color with both your dominant and non-dominant hand.

Day Forty-one

- Drink seven glasses of water and three cups of green tea.
- Walk for at least 15 minutes this morning and 15 minutes this afternoon.
- Go to a quiet space, sit comfortably, close your eyes, take deep breaths and focus only on the air flowing into your nose, down into your lungs, and back out for 5 minutes.
- Stand on one leg for 15 seconds, and then the other for 15 seconds.

Brain activities:

- Put your hands together. Move your hands in a figure 8 motion in front of your body while marching in place. While your body is in motion, say your favorite dessert out loud. Spell it forward. Spell it backward. How many letters does the word have? Does your telephone number contain that number? If yes, say the section of your phone number that contains that number. Repeat the answer backwards. If no, repeat any section of your phone number backwards. This exercise should be done with a partner who can ask you the questions.
- Solve these problems in your head.

$215 \times 2 =$ ___ $31 + 53 =$ ___ $194 - 63 =$ ___ $75/5 =$ ___

- Make a bucket list.

Day Forty-two

- Drink seven glasses of water and three cups of green tea.
- Walk for at least 15 minutes this morning and 15 minutes this afternoon.
- Go to a quiet space, sit comfortably, close your eyes, take deep breaths and focus only on the air flowing into your nose, down into your lungs, and back out for 5 minutes.
- Stand on one leg for 15 seconds, and then the other for 15 seconds.

Brain activities:

- March in place while rubbing your belly in a circular motion with your dominant hand, alternate touching your left and right ears with your non-dominant hand while singing the Twinkle Twinkle Little Star.
- Solve these problems in your head.

$285 \times 2 = $ ___ $194 + 51 = $ ___ $612 - 47 = $ ___ $126/2 = $ ___

- Make every animal sound you can think of out loud. Laugh. Spell the names of the animals and their sounds out loud. Forwards and backwards.

Day Forty-three

- Drink seven glasses of water and three cups of green tea.
- Walk for at least 15 minutes this morning and 15 minutes this afternoon.
- Go to a quiet space, sit comfortably, close your eyes, take deep breaths and focus only on the air flowing into your nose, down into your lungs, and back out for 5 minutes.
- Stand on one leg for 15 seconds, and then the other for 15 seconds.

Brain activities:

- While marching in place and doing arm circles at the same time, think of a day you spent at the mall. How many people went with you? How long ago did you go? Was the mall busy? Did you have to wait in any lines? What did you buy?
- Crumple up ten sheets of paper and aim for a basket/box. See how many you can get in with your dominant hand. See how many you can get in with your non-dominant hand. Repeat with your eyes closed.
- Divide the year you were born by the day you were born. Multipy that number by the month you were born.

Day Forty-four

- Drink seven glasses of water and three cups of green tea.
- Walk for at least 15 minutes this morning and 15 minutes this afternoon.
- Go to a quiet space, sit comfortably, close your eyes, take deep breaths and focus only on the air flowing into your nose, down into your lungs, and back out for 5 minutes.
- Stand on one leg for 15 seconds, and then the other for 15 seconds.

Brain activities:

- Eat with your non-dominant hand today.
- Sing Head, Shoulders, Knees, and Toes. Head, shoulders, knees, and toes, Knees and toes. Head, shoulders, knees, and toes, Knees and toes. Eyes and ears and mouth and nose. Head, shoulders, knees, and toes, Knees and toes!
- Sing it in Spanish. Cabeza (head), hombros (shoulders), rodillas (knees) y (and) dedos (toes), rodillas y dedos. Cabeza, hombros, rodillas y dedos, rodillas y dedos. Ojos (eyes) y (and) orejas (ears) y boca (mouth) y nariz (nose). Cabeza, hombros, rodillas y dedos, rodillas y dedos!

Day Forty-five

- Drink seven glasses of water and three cups of green tea.
- Walk for at least 15 minutes this morning and 15 minutes this afternoon.
- Go to a quiet space, sit comfortably, close your eyes, take deep breaths and focus only on the air flowing into your nose, down into your lungs, and back out for 5 minutes.
- Stand on one leg for 15 seconds, and then the other for 15 seconds.

Brain activities:
- Juggle with scarves today while singing Happy Birthday, the alphabet, or your national anthem.
- Play a board game.
- Learn the words for rooms of your house in either Spanish or French. To help with memorization write down the words and place them in each room.

	Spanish	French
Bedroom	el dormitorio	chambre
Kitchen	la cocina	cuisine
Bathroom	baño	salle de bains
Living Room	sala	salon
Dining Room	el comedor	salle à manger

Day Forty-six

- Drink seven glasses of water and three cups of green tea.
- Walk for at least 15 minutes this morning and 15 minutes this afternoon.
- Go to a quiet space, sit comfortably, close your eyes, take deep breaths and focus only on the air flowing into your nose, down into your lungs, and back out for 5 minutes.
- Stand on one leg for 15 seconds, and then the other for 15 seconds.

Brain activities:

- Alternate moving one side of your body with the other (ex. lunges, leg kicks or tap your toes) while clapping your hands. Say a different city every time you move the right side of your body. Say a different state every time you move the left side. Perform this exercise for at least one minute.
- Sing Twinkle, Twinkle, Little Star. Write down the words. Now keep the tune, but replace all of the words with something relating to your own life. For example, shiny, shiny, coffee cup...Write them down.

Day Forty-seven

- Drink seven glasses of water and three cups of green tea.
- Walk for at least 15 minutes this morning and 15 minutes this afternoon.
- Go to a quiet space, sit comfortably, close your eyes, take deep breaths and focus only on the air flowing into your nose, down into your lungs, and back out for 5 minutes.
- Stand on one leg for 15 seconds, and then the other for 15 seconds.

Brain activities:

- Brush your teeth with your non-dominant hand.
- Keep a piece of paper handy today. Keep track of all of your steps manually, no fitness trackers. If you walk to the bathroom, count the steps, write them down. The kitchen? Same thing. Add them up at the end of the day. Divide them by the number of hours you have been awake. How many steps did you average per hour?

Day Forty-eight

- Drink seven glasses of water and three cups of green tea.
- Walk for at least 15 minutes this morning and 15 minutes this afternoon.
- Go to a quiet space, sit comfortably, close your eyes, take deep breaths and focus only on the air flowing into your nose, down into your lungs, and back out for 5 minutes.
- Stand on one leg for 15 seconds, and then the other for 15 seconds.

Brain activities:

- Put your hands together. Move your hands in a figure 8 motion in front of your body while marching in place. While your body is in motion, say your favorite TV show out loud. Spell it forward. Spell it backward. How many letters does the word have? Does your telephone number contain that number? If yes, say the section of your phone number that contains that number. Repeat the answer backwards. If no, repeat any section of your phone number backwards. This exercise should be done with a partner who can ask you the questions.
- Count how many windows in your home. Multiply that number by the number of doors in your home.
- Count how many cupboards are in your home. Multiply that number by the number of rooms in your home.
- Count how many lightbulbs are in your home. Divide that number by the number of appliances you have in your home.

Day Forty-nine

- Drink seven glasses of water and three cups of green tea.
- Walk for at least 15 minutes this morning and 15 minutes this afternoon.
- Go to a quiet space, sit comfortably, close your eyes, take deep breaths and focus only on the air flowing into your nose, down into your lungs, and back out for 5 minutes.
- Stand on one leg for 15 seconds, and then the other for 15 seconds.

Brain activities:

- March in place while rubbing your belly in a circular motion with your dominant hand, alternate touching your left and right ears with your non-dominant hand while singing the alphabet backwards.
- Estimate how many calories you eat on a daily basis.
- Carbohydrates should make up 45-65% of your caloric intake. Carbohydrates provide 4 calories per gram, determine your recommended intake by taking 45-65% of your total daily caloric intake and then dividing that number by 4.
- Fat should make up 20-35% of your caloric intake. Fats provide 9 calories per gram, determine your recommended intake by taking 20-35% of your total daily caloric intake and then dividing that number by 9.
- Protein should make up 15-35% of your caloric intake. Protein provides 4 calories per gram, determine your recommended intake by taking 15-35% of your total daily caloric intake and then dividing that number by 4.

Day Fifty

- Drink seven glasses of water and three cups of green tea.
- Walk for at least 15 minutes this morning and 15 minutes this afternoon.
- Go to a quiet space, sit comfortably, close your eyes, take deep breaths and focus only on the air flowing into your nose, down into your lungs, and back out for 5 minutes.
- Stand on one leg for 15 seconds, and then the other for 15 seconds.

Brain activities:

- While marching in place and doing arm circles, think of your favorite memory. What is it? When did it occur? Who was with you? Can you remember what you were wearing? What was the weather like that day?
- Solve these problems in your head.

$231 \times 6 =$ ___ $116 + 75 =$ ___ $781 - 124 =$ ___ $165/5 =$ ___

- How many words can you make with the following letters:

C K I W L

- Name 3 cities that begin with the letter P.
- Work on memorizing the capitals of the fifty United States this week.

Alabama - Montgomery	Colorado - Denver
Alaska - Juneau	Connecticut - Hartford
Arizona - Phoenix	Delaware - Dover
Arkansas - Little Rock	Florida - Tallahasee
California - Sacramento	Georgia - Atlanta

Day Fifty-one

- Drink seven glasses of water and three cups of green tea.
- Walk for at least 15 minutes this morning and 15 minutes this afternoon.
- Go to a quiet space, sit comfortably, close your eyes, take deep breaths and focus only on the air flowing into your nose, down into your lungs, and back out for 5 minutes.
- Stand on one leg for 15 seconds, and then the other for 15 seconds.

Brain activities:

- Eat with your non-dominant hand today.
- Solve these problems in your head.

$771 \times 2 =$ ___ $541 + 332 =$ ___ $851 - 227 =$ ___ $144/12 =$ ___

- How many words can you make with the following letters:

O O L N E

- Say and spell all of the days of the week out loud. Now spell them backwards.
- Read everything out loud today.
- Work on memorizing the capitals of the fifty United States this week.

Hawaii - Honolulu

Idaho - Boise

Illinois - Springfield

Indiana - Indianapolis

Iowa - Des Moines

Kansas - Topeka

Kentucky - Frankfort

Louisiana - Baton Rouge

Maine - Augusta

Maryland - Annapolis

Day Fifty-two

- Drink seven glasses of water and three cups of green tea.
- Walk for at least 15 minutes this morning and 15 minutes this afternoon.
- Go to a quiet space, sit comfortably, close your eyes, take deep breaths and focus only on the air flowing into your nose, down into your lungs, and back out for 5 minutes.
- Stand on one leg for 15 seconds, and then the other for 15 seconds.

Brain activities:

- Time to juggle with scarves. Count each time you throw a scarf. How high can you get?
- Solve these problems in your head.

354 x 2 = ___   681 + 93 = ___   872 - 437 = ___   95/19 = ___

- How many words can you make with the following letters:

R G E T A

- Name the 3 states that start with the letter N.
- When you were a kid where did you want to live when you grew up?
- Work on memorizing the capitals of the fifty United States this week.

Massachusetts - Boston	Montana - Helena
Michigan - Lansing	Nebraska - Omaha
Minnesota - Saint Paul	Nevada - Carson City
Mississippi - Jackson	New Hampshire - Concord
Missouri - Jefferson City	New Jersey - Trenton

Day Fifty-three

- Drink seven glasses of water and three cups of green tea.
- Walk for at least 15 minutes this morning and 15 minutes this afternoon.
- Go to a quiet space, sit comfortably, close your eyes, take deep breaths and focus only on the air flowing into your nose, down into your lungs, and back out for 5 minutes.
- Stand on one leg for 15 seconds, and then the other for 15 seconds.

Brain activities:

- Alternate moving one side of your body with the other (ex. lunges, leg kicks or tap your toes) while clapping your hands. Say a different letter every time you move the right side of your body. Say a different number every time you move the left side. Perform this exercise for at least one minute.
- Solve these problems in your head.

$50 \times 13 =$ ___ $120 + 941 =$ ___ $166 - 148 =$ ___ $52/4 =$ ___

- How many words can you make with the following letters:

F S T R I

- Work on memorizing the capitals of the fifty United States this week.

New Mexico - Santa Fe	Oklahoma - Oklahoma City
New York - Albany	Oregon - Salem
North Carolina - Raleigh	Pennsylvania - Harrisburg
North Dakota - Ohio	Rhode Island - Providence
Ohio - Columbus	South Carolina - Columbia

Day Fifty-four

- Drink seven glasses of water and three cups of green tea.
- Walk for at least 15 minutes this morning and 15 minutes this afternoon.
- Go to a quiet space, sit comfortably, close your eyes, take deep breaths and focus only on the air flowing into your nose, down into your lungs, and back out for 5 minutes.
- Stand on one leg for 15 seconds, and then the other for 15 seconds.

Brain activities:

- Brush your teeth with your non-dominant hand.
- Solve these problems in your head.

$161 \times 6 =$ ___ $387 + 25 =$ ___ $321 - 113 =$ ___ $608/4 =$ ___

- How many words can you make with the following letters:

$$Y \ E \ T \ S \ A$$

- Name the 7 continents. Spell them out loud forwards and backwards.
- Work on memorizing the capitals of the fifty United States this week.

South Dakota - Pierre

Tennessee - Nashville

Texas - Austin

Utah - Salt Lake City

Vermont - Montpelier

Virginia - Richmond

Washington - Olympia

West Virginia - Charleston

Wisconsin - Madison

Wyoming - Cheyenne

Day Fifty-five

- Drink seven glasses of water and three cups of green tea.
- Walk for at least 15 minutes this morning and 15 minutes this afternoon.
- Go to a quiet space, sit comfortably, close your eyes, take deep breaths and focus only on the air flowing into your nose, down into your lungs, and back out for 5 minutes.
- Stand on one leg for 15 seconds, and then the other for 15 seconds.

Brain activities:

- Put your hands together. Move your hands in a figure 8 motion in front of your body while marching in place. While your body is in motion, say your favorite day of the week out loud. Spell it forward. Spell it backward. How many letters does the word have? Does your telephone number contain that number? If yes, say the section of your phone number that contains that number. Repeat the answer backwards. If no, repeat any section of your phone number backwards. This exercise should be done with a partner who can ask you the questions.
- Solve these problems in your head.

$12 + 13 + 14 + 5 =$ ___ $98 - 9 - 8 - 4 - 2 - 1 =$ ___

- How many words can you make with the following letters:

S E H A R

- Write down as many countries as you know. Spell them forwards and backwards out loud.
- What did you eat for dinner four days ago? What did you eat for lunch three days ago?
- Continue to work on memorizing the fifty United States.

Day Fifty-six

- Drink seven glasses of water and three cups of green tea.
- Walk for at least 15 minutes this morning and 15 minutes this afternoon.
- Go to a quiet space, sit comfortably, close your eyes, take deep breaths and focus only on the air flowing into your nose, down into your lungs, and back out for 5 minutes.
- Stand on one leg for 15 seconds, and then the other for 15 seconds.

Brain activities:

- March in place while rubbing your belly in a circular motion with your dominant hand, alternate touching your left and right ears with your non-dominant hand while singing Mary Had a Little Lamb.
- Solve these problems in your head.

$21 + 31 + 41 + 6 =$ ___ $56 - 1 - 8 - 4 - 7 - 9 =$ ___

- How many words can you make with the following letters:

G I E K N

- Name 3 politicians past or present with first or last names that start with the letter A.
- How many people do you know were born in February?
- Continue to work on memorizing the fifty United States.

Day Fifty-seven

- Drink seven glasses of water and three cups of green tea.
- Walk for at least 15 minutes this morning and 15 minutes this afternoon.
- Go to a quiet space, sit comfortably, close your eyes, take deep breaths and focus only on the air flowing into your nose, down into your lungs, and back out for 5 minutes.
- Stand on one leg for 20 seconds, and then the other for 20 seconds.

Brain activities:

- While marching in place and doing arm circles, think of your favorite vacation. Where did you go? When did it occur? Who was with you? What was the weather like? What was your favorite part?
- Using a pencil and paper, draw a chair, a swing set, and an airplane with your dominant hand. Then draw the same pictures with your non-dominant hand.
- Count how many beds in your home. Multiply that number by the number of pillows in your home.
- Count how many bowls are in your home. Multiply that number by the number of spoons in your home.
- Count how many plates are in your home. Multiply that number by the number of forks you have in your home.

Day Fifty-eight

- Drink seven glasses of water and three cups of green tea.
- Walk for at least 15 minutes this morning and 15 minutes this afternoon.
- Go to a quiet space, sit comfortably, close your eyes, take deep breaths and focus only on the air flowing into your nose, down into your lungs, and back out for 5 minutes.
- Stand on one leg for 20 seconds, and then the other for 20 seconds.

Brain activities:

- Eat with your non-dominant hand today.
- Solve these problems in your head.

$22 + 33 + 44 + 6 =$ ___ $68 - 2 - 7 - 3 - 6 - 8 =$ ___

- Read everything out loud today.
- Learn the words for items in your house in either Spanish or French. To help with memorization write down the words and place them nearby the items.

	Spanish	French
Window	la ventana	la fenêtre
Couch	la sofá	le canapé
Bed	la cama	le lit
Towel	la toalla	la serviette
Cup	la taza	la tasse

Day Fifty-Nine

- Drink seven glasses of water and three cups of green tea.
- Walk for at least 15 minutes this morning and 15 minutes this afternoon.
- Go to a quiet space, sit comfortably, close your eyes, take deep breaths and focus only on the air flowing into your nose, down into your lungs, and back out for 5 minutes.
- Stand on one leg for 20 seconds, and then the other for 20 seconds.

Brain activities:

- Time to juggle with scarves. Say the alphabet backwards while juggling.
- Solve these problems in your head.

$39 + 3 + 102 + 6 =$ ___ $88 - 13 - 7 - 3 - 6 =$ ___

- Sing Happy Birthday. Write down the words. Now keep the tune, but replace all of the words with something relating to your own life. For example, It's so co-old outside…Write them down.
- Say and spell all of the months of the year out loud.
- Brush your teeth with your non-dominant hand today.

Day Sixty

- Drink seven glasses of water and three cups of green tea.
- Walk for at least 15 minutes this morning and 15 minutes this afternoon.
- Go to a quiet space, sit comfortably, close your eyes, take deep breaths and focus only on the air flowing into your nose, down into your lungs, and back out for 5 minutes.
- Stand on one leg for 20 seconds, and then the other for 20 seconds.

Brain activities:

- Alternate moving one side of your body with the other (ex. lunges, leg kicks or tap your toes) while clapping your hands. Say a different person's first name every time you move the right side of your body. Say a different person's last name every time you move the left side. Perform this exercise for at least one minute.
- Keep a piece of paper handy today. Keep track of the number of times you say 3 certain words today. Such as time, now, and where. Multiply the amounts at the end of the day. Then divide them by 3.
- Test yourself today. How many states can you remember? How many capitals can you remember?

Day Sixty-one & Beyond

Continue to:

- Drink seven glasses of water and three cups of green tea every day.
- Walk for at least 15 minutes in the morning and 15 minutes in the afternoon.
- Go to a quiet space, sit comfortably, close your eyes, take deep breaths and focus only on the air flowing into your nose, down into your lungs, and back out for 5 minutes every day.
- Stand on one leg for 20 seconds, and then the other for 20 seconds every day, working your way to 30 seconds when you are ready.

Brain activities:

Take a sheet of paper, cut it into 60 pieces and number them from 1 to 60. Put the pieces in a bowl and mix them around. Each morning grab out a number and do the brain activities for that day. So, if you pull out the number 37, go to Day 37 and do the brain activities. When the activities from this book become easy and routine, be proud of yourself and move on. Challenge yourself by learning a new language, playing a new instrument, or starting a new hobby, but please stick with the water and green tea; walking in the morning and afternoon; meditation; and the balance exercise.

www.ingramcontent.com/pod-product-compliance
Lightning Source LLC
Chambersburg PA
CBHW050515290526
45786CB00007B/2572